for LIFE

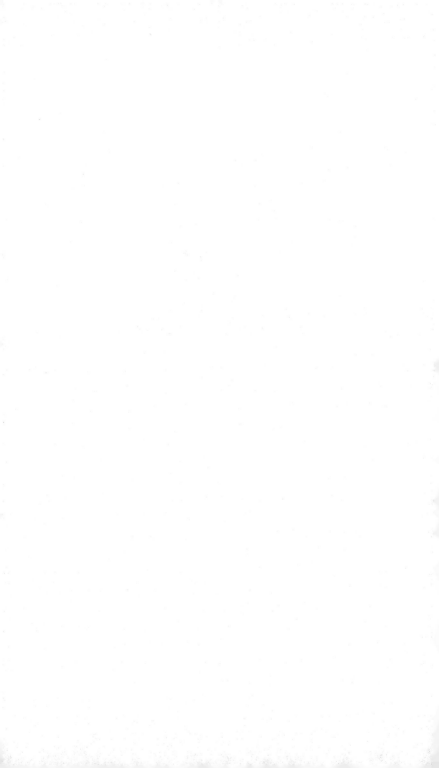

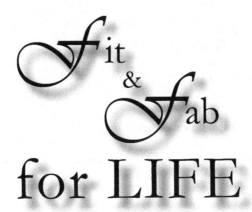

Fit & Fab for LIFE

50 MOTIVATIONAL TIPS TO HELP YOU
GET FIT AND BE FABULOUS FOR LIFE

FRANCYNE WALKER

authorHOUSE®

AuthorHouse™
1663 Liberty Drive
Bloomington, IN 47403
www.authorhouse.com
Phone: 1-800-839-8640

© 2013 by Francyne Walker. All rights reserved.

No part of this book may be reproduced, stored in a retrieval system, or transmitted
by any means without the written permission of the author.

Published by AuthorHouse   02/28/2013

ISBN: 978-1-4772-9837-4 (sc)
ISBN: 978-1-4772-9836-7 (e)

Library of Congress Control Number: 2012923471

Any people depicted in stock imagery provided by Thinkstock are models,
and such images are being used for illustrative purposes only.
Certain stock imagery © Thinkstock.

This book is printed on acid-free paper.

Because of the dynamic nature of the Internet, any web addresses or links
contained in this book may have changed since publication and may no longer be
valid. The views expressed in this work are solely those of the author and do not
necessarily reflect the views of the publisher, and the publisher hereby disclaims
any responsibility for them.

Contents

This book is dedicated to my family and
the memory of my mother, Vivian Walker,
who was a fighter to the end.

I'll always love you Ma!

Introduction

I've always been weight conscious, but on this particular occasion I had picked up more weight than I wanted to carry, sometimes at least 15 pounds. This weight gain occurred after a major a breakup, coupled with my life feeling out of sync. This was around 2008. As an emotional eater, I tended to respond with food by comforting myself in the midst of a crisis. I remembered deciding to have foot surgery, two bunionectomies back to back, which basically grounded me for about six months where I was not as mobile as I could be. This contributed to additional weight gain as I remembered experiencing a deeper sense of hopelessness more than any other time in my life. It wasn't until I went back to work and realized I needed to focus on doing what I love and make a transition in my career. At the end of 2008, the company I worked for offered a voluntary buyout and as sure as I know my name I knew this was

Francyne Walker

an opportunity that I couldn't pass up. It was one of the best decisions I made in my life. So in 2009, I set out to complete my master's degree, lose the weight I gained during my recuperation period following surgery, and pursue my dreams of a broadcasting career.

I'll admit, I never planned on writing a book about weight loss, but sometimes the best things in life aren't always planned. *Fit and Fab for Life* came as a result of being asked the question so many times, following my weight loss, "How are you going to keep it off?" I was rather puzzled by the question although it made sense. Only one in six people keep their weight off according to research from the Penn State College of Medicine. One cannot argue that your attitude is paramount to permanent weight loss. Therefore being "fit and fab" is more a philosophy, a state of mind, hence a state of being. I outline several tips that collectively provide a breeding ground for a positive attitude. Although I lost 60 pounds with the help of a program, I don't tout one specific diet program over another. The kind of diet program you choose should be based on your lifestyle and preferences based on your personality. This will also enable you to stay committed and hence be successful. I wanted to encourage not only myself, but also anyone one else that's on this interesting, but rewarding journey and congratulate those who are moving to the next phase of the journey—maintenance. I have successfully kept 60 pounds off for a year and I continue to work on maintaining that loss, staying fit and being fab for life. It is my hope that you will laugh a little, and begin to apply one, some or all these tips so you can join the Fit and Fab for Life revolution.

1

What's Up Doc?

While reading this book does not require you to check with your physician, you should definitely check with them before beginning a weight loss and/or exercise program. Additionally, one cannot be fit and fabulous by avoiding regular checkups that help us ensure everything is in order. Mammograms, physicals, dental and vision checkups, and pap smears are necessary to stay in tip-top shape from the inside out. Knowledge is power and avoiding those routine check-ups will not protect you from bad news. It will actually empower you. Going to the doctor enables you to be proactive in light of the results. A lot of diseases and ailments are preventable if we make wiser decisions when it comes to our health. Avoiding the doctor puts you in a more vulnerable position and it doesn't empower you to manage your health. Of course if you're starting a fitness program, you should consult with your physician for a routine physical. There are basic

Francyne Walker

exams and tests everyone should have and then there are specific tests one should have based on an assessment of their health. Saying "What's Up Doc?" on a regular basis goes a long way in staying fit and fab. Taking care of yourself should not exclude the care and consultation from your regular doctor. What you learn will not hurt you, but will definitely help you be in a better position to deal with your health.

2

Make Mine a Double

Working out two times a day is not uncommon, especially if you're trying to reach your weight loss goals quicker. If you're short on time, you can probably do 30 minutes in the morning and 30 minutes or an hour later in the day or when it's more convenient for you. While I don't do it on a daily basis, every now and then I usually choose a day where I may do two separate workouts in one day. I might even do an hour of strength training in the morning and an hour of cardio in the afternoon. This is particularly good if you want to maximize your workouts, but may not have a two hour block of time to devote at one time. Even if you work out for a half hour on any particular day due to time constraints, it still counts as time spent moving your body. The point is that you give it your best effort and don't feel pressured to work out two times in one day until your body has become used to working out regularly. Even if you may even elect to exercise one day a week where you do two sessions, that's sufficient. Just don't overdo it. Breaking it up sometimes is okay if you stay committed to your exercise schedule.

3

Keep it Simple

It is a lot easier to maintain a more regimented diet through the week versus the weekend where the days are less structured. Preparation and planning are key factors for staying on track. I find that cooking in bulk eliminates the need to impulsively reach for fast food to feed your hunger. A typical scenario we can all relate to is getting off work with a ravenous appetite and having to stop by the grocery store on the way home. This is setting you up for potential temptation. Brown-bagging your lunch is essential to your success as well. I usually pre-cook chicken breasts and turkey burgers to have on hand for lunch and dinner. Then I'm able to include them in soups, salads or entrees. There are so many different combos of turkey burger sandwiches that you can experiment with different vegetable toppings and condiments. It really is up to you and this is a quick way to get your vegetable servings as well as protein. When going out to dinner, check restaurant menus online so that you're not caught by surprise at the restaurant. Then you can pre-plan what you will order when you get there. I find it easier to stay on point with simple fare as it also encourages clean eating, minus heavy sauces and creams, which in most cases, can be fattening. Consider experimenting with your food for variety's sake. You don't have to be committed to the same food the same way, although I find it easier when I'm really busy to pre-cook food and have it on hand. Find recipes that make chicken breasts in various ways as well to keep from getting bored with your dishes.

4

Change Your Flock

⸺⬦⸺

If you surround yourself around people who like to overeat, it will be hard to resist the influence of the group. Plus, you'll be hard pressed to exercise willpower. You'll eventually justify why you're overeating and negotiate with yourself that you'll work it off later. If you put yourself in a position where you are surrounded by healthy foods and healthy-minded people, you will more than likely eat healthy as well as make healthier lifestyle choices. Surrounding yourself with people who are weight-conscious will no doubt have an influence on what you do. If you strictly hang around "chili cheese fry" friends, chances are you will make "chili cheese fry" choices. I am not suggesting that you totally abandon your friends, or family for that matter, and never indulge in chili cheese fries again. However, a slight change in your flock will do wonders to enable a successful weight loss journey. Start setting the barometer for your friends to lead healthier lives by suggesting alternative activities that help the group get healthier. Rather than indulging at your favorite restaurant on a regular basis, hire a trainer or a dance instructor to train you and your friends for that night. Encourage everyone to bring healthy dishes to share afterwards. You just have to be vigilant about your weight loss goals and ultimately your weight maintenance goals. Taking different exercise classes will also help you make new friends and build relationships with people who are fitness-minded. You can start your own circle of people by being a positive influence in others' lives. Keep in mind, you don't have to do this alone. Find a community, create a community, and become a community where maintaining healthy living is the norm and not the exception.

5

You Better Work It

I can almost hear RuPaul's voice somewhere saying "You better work it, honey!" There are so many "diets" to choose from when it comes to taking the pounds off. The truth is any "diet" can work if you work it. Now, I'm not advocating fad diets or anything that causes you to take drastic or harmful meatures but the key is to choose a weight loss program that fits your lifestyle. You have to find an eating program that will be easy for you to endure for the long haul. Some people are more comfortable with prepared meals delivered to their doorstep while others are more comfortable preparing their own meals. If counting calories, or points and crunching numbers is your thing, go for it. Either way, you have to be committed to your program. Don't give up and if you fall off the wagon, just get back on. When my mom got sick, I totally fell off the wagon for about three months. Once she was out of the woods, I got right back on the program when I was able to focus more on myself. Although I was not following my original eating plan, I kept on exercising so that my weight loss efforts weren't totally lost. So whatever weight loss program you choose, it will have its share of challenges, but you just have to work it honey!

6

Let's Switch

———◆———

Your cardio may consist of a daily run or exercising on your favorite machine—treadmill, stepper or elliptical trainer. Ideally, it's best to switch it up so your body doesn't get used to doing one thing. Variety is necessary to staying motivated and not becoming bored. I admit I bore easily when it comes to cardio machines so what I do sometimes is do 10 minute stretches on a machine and then I'll go to a weight machine. I'll increase the intensity every time I get back on the elliptical machine or the treadmill until I have done a total hour of cardio. Switching up allows you to try new exercises to see what you like. I don't like the stationary bike, but I love spinning—a fast-paced class where you're riding the bike while being guided by the instructor to increase the tension of the ride and the music is extremely high energy. It's a great interval exercise. Trying something different like a Zumba dance class or water aerobics breaks the monotony of an everyday cardio routine. For example, I eat cold bran cereal for breakfast just about every day, but sometimes I'll have a vegetarian omelet just to break the monotony. Try warm cereal, like oatmeal, complete with nuts, dried fruit and brown sugar. Add lime to your water instead of lemon. You get the picture? Throwing in a slight variation, here and there, keeps you from getting bored.

7

Say "Cheese" and "Thank You"

When some people praise your weight loss, they just don't seem to stop there. Sometimes, they use the compliment as an opportunity to tell you not to lose more weight. Never mind, they're usually in a place where they could stand to lose a few pounds themselves, but they want to gauge your weight loss. I've come to realize why people do it because your weight loss seems to hold a mirror up to them that sometimes convict them. I'm not making generalizations, but this is one of the reasons why people will seemingly dole out "good" advice about not "getting too skinny." The truth is it's a lot easier to direct someone else than it is to tackle your weight issue. Let me say this loud and clear, "Your personal best is personal." It's absolutely nobody's business because you know where you want to be as far as your weight loss goals are concerned. If you look in the mirror and you feel like you're not where you want to be, then change it. You are the captain of your ship, steer it where you want to. It doesn't matter what's in, thick or thin, just be comfortable in your own skin. Now, it does feel good to have people notice and applaud your efforts, just understand that you are not obligated to dialogue with them or defend your weight loss goals. Applause and positive comments are great but you are in this for the long haul and self-motivation is key to maintaining your ideal weight. So smile, say "thank you" and keep it moving.

8

The Great Closet Makeover

At my current weight, I wear everything from a size 4 to a size 10, depending on the designer and the cut. When I was 215 pounds, I wore everything from a size 14 to a size 18. Ouch! I still cringe when I type that number, but it's the truth anyhow. People have jokingly told me to hold on to those clothes just in case I gain any weight back. Come to think of it, maybe they were serious because for those that have lost weight, keeping old clothes, in my opinion, can sabotage your new way of doing things. That's the worst advice because frankly I don't want to ever wear those black pants again. I wore them three days a week because I refused to buy a bunch of clothes in that size range. The only reminders you need are old photos and maybe a few select items to remind you to stay focused on maintaining the new you.

Francyne Walker

9

Keep It Moving

Constipation can be a pain in the "you know what." Look, can we talk? I've heard many unfortunate stories where people have bowel movements maybe once a week and they think it's normal. Newsflash: It's not! Bowel movements should be a regular occurrence, at least two to three times a day. Getting a good colon cleanse on a regular basis is a good idea to help facilitate the flow of things. A diet high in fiber and drinking lots of water is an important component of bowel regularity as well. It's not a pretty subject and it can be a little gross, but colorectal cancer and colon cancer are not pretty subjects you want to be forced to discuss either. So, keep it moving shugga. I promise you, feeling light and breezy compared to feeling weighed down and full of crap is for the birds.

10

Weigh In Often

I weigh myself every morning after I wake up. I thank God for another day and I move forward with the day. I don't always take the number too seriously (and I have) because a minor spike could simply mean the result of a high salt diet the night before. This spike might be a pound or a half a pound and may disappear in a day or so. If I go more than three pounds over my ideal weight, I'm on it. This two-three pound spike could also be due to a more indulgent weekend but it's important to get right back on track and work to lose the weight. The clinic that I go to prefers that I weigh in weekly. I also try and weigh in weekly as much as possible to stay on top of my goal and remain accountable to people who help me get back to it right away. So weigh in often and don't get overworked about the tiny spikes in weight gain. There's no need to panic, just get busy and watch your intake for the week and maintain. Use these spikes as a guide to steer you back towards your ideal weight. It's a constant effort, but the rewards of maintaining your weight far outweigh the efforts. Think about it, even if you decided to never lose weight and you're happy where you are, you still have to watch your weight so that you stay where you are. Trust me, I know it can be a struggle at times with a hectic lifestyle, but you can do it.

11

Love Your Kitchen

———— ❖ ————

Fast food choices can sabotage the best efforts when it comes to losing weight. Clean eating is where you have the best success. Chicken, fish, vegetables minus heavy creams or sauces are best and eliminate consumption of extra calories. The catch is you will have to prepare these foods yourself, so learn to love your kitchen. Buy nice cook wear and utensils. Places like Home Goods and TJ Maxx have a variety of nice items to make cooking more enjoyable. Stock your kitchen with healthy staples that you can reach for to prepare quick meals. Experiment with different vegetables and seasonings to keep your palate dancing. I love stir-fries because it allows me to throw a ton of different vegetables together with chicken, fish or beef and create a "kitchen sink" stir fry. It's an easy way to try a different variety combo of vegetables. I love dining out but the success of weight loss was attributed more to preparing my own meals versus going out to eat all the time. Preparing things like grilled chicken breasts ahead of time will go a long way in helping you resist the visit to your favorite drive-thru all the time. Having this one ingredient will enable you to make delicious dishes like chicken tacos, chicken salad, grilled chicken salad, and chicken soup. If you feel like you're going to burp a feather, switch it up. To tell you to never dine out is unrealistic. Get into the practice of preparing meals for yourself and really loving this process and watch the extra pounds and money you'll save.

12

See the Big Picture

Buy a full-length mirror to appreciate who you are now and who you are becoming. It helps when getting dressed to have a full-length mirror to see the big picture of how you look head-to-toe. You don't have to spend a lot of money for a mirror either. It certainly beats the mirror on the dresser which usually cuts you off at the waist, not allowing you to appreciate yourself full-length. You cannot underestimate the value of the big picture. After all, it's only more fabulousness staring back at you. Imagine being able to always walk out the door looking your best because you were able to tweak your outfit as a result of being able to see yourself head-to-toe. Whether it was changing your shoes or eliminating visible bulges or panty lines, all this can be accomplished by doing a once-over in the mirror beforehand.

Francyne Walker

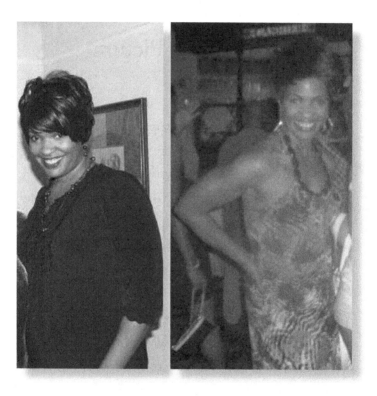

Me, Before and After

13

Eat It, Write It

This is probably one of the most tedious, but most effective ways to stay on top of your weight loss efforts. Writing down what you eat helps you see exactly what you're doing and how it affects your efforts. Grabbing a handful of this or just a pinch of that can add up and sabotage you. It helped me stay on top of my diet program that had been set up for me. You can use an actual food journal that keeps track of your exercise activity as well or you can buy a tiny notebook and write down everything you eat. Myfitnesspal.com allows you to track your food, calories and exercise. If you're often on the go, a tiny notebook may suffice. I prefer a food journal because I can just put my food choices for the day in the appropriate boxes for breakfast, lunch, dinner and snacks. The most important thing is to get into the habit of writing down what you eat. Sometimes it's a challenge and if you skip a day, start fresh the next day.

14

Embrace the New Normal

Some people don't like the word "diet" but actually what you eat every day is basically considered your diet. Changing the way you eat for a period of time is usually what people associate "diet" with. You diet and exercise to lose weight and then you go back to your normal routine. But then, think about it, isn't the old normal what caused you to get to where you are today? You're embarking on a journey to change your body for the better. So embrace the new normal and whatever that means for you. If drinking 64 ounces of water, working out five to six days a week or writing down your food intake are your new habits, then stick with them. Your new normal is what will help the lifestyle changes become permanent habits.

15

Spare the Splurge

————◦◉◦————

When I was dieting to lose weight, I rarely had dessert as the program I followed did not allow me to satisfy my sweet tooth. If I went out to dinner, I stuck with the predictable—a grilled chicken salad as I knew my weight would fluctuate greatly if I deviated from the plan. I wanted to see the scale go down continuously versus sliding back and forth. Whether it's a glass of wine or a piece of cake, try to refrain from indulging too much with those treats to ensure your weight is on a continual downward spiral. If you must celebrate a special occasion, go ahead, but make sure you do a little extra cardio at the gym. Just don't get in the habit of splurging all the time as it slows down your progress and it will only frustrate you.

16

Get a Jump Start

---◦◉◦---

The "lemonade" diet, the cabbage soup diet, the baby food diet all promise rapid weight loss yet they seem like drastic measures that will test even people with the strongest willpower. A lot of programs out there do offer a way to follow a more specific diet that includes all food groups to allow you to lose a certain amount of weight in a given period. I like to think of this as an initial incentive to get started and stick with it. Losing just a little weight will make you feel like a million bucks so cherish this tiny accomplishment while you continue on your weight loss journey.

The program I followed started with a cleansing phase in which I lost about five pounds in three days. This was a drop in a bucket compared to the 60 pounds that I wanted to lose, but it was a nice motivator for the long journey ahead. Just be sensible in your goals and the approaches you take because at the end of the day it's about being healthy while losing weight. Weight loss through safe, yet drastic, measures can just what the doctor ordered to get you going.

17

What's Eating You?

Oftentimes our lives can be spinning out of control and we feel helpless in the midst of what seems like a tornado. Instead of tackling what's eating us or making us unhappy, we reach for a drug that feels good and tastes good—food. The obesity rates are a clear indication that food is a popular drug of choice. Maybe, we feel like we have no control over our circumstances, but we certainly have control over that chocolate cake on the plate. This can give us a sense of temporary empowerment or a numbing effect to what's going on inside of us. Trust me, been there, done that and I. LOVE. CHOCOLATE. I am an emotional eater and in the past I've responded to "life happens" with poor food choices. I was in a dead-end job, not fulfilling my dreams of a broadcasting career and entertaining toxic relationships. Once I took responsibility for changing my situation, I was able to assess situations differently and choose food for nourishment purposes.

I am a big proponent of counseling and if you need to consult someone, do it. This will help you address what's eating you and then make "your best life" choices according to what you've learned about yourself and your situation. This is a continual journey that requires you to check in with yourself regularly through prayer and meditation.

18

Play Dress Up

———————————•◉•———————————

Whether I was a size 16 or a size 8, I always liked dressing up except I refused to buy a whole new wardrobe of clothes in my former size. I always believed I wouldn't be that size forever and as I lost weight, I was able to wear clothes that were hanging in my closet. I wanted to go shopping again after my confidence grew, knowing that I would be able to find things that fit. So, go shopping and try on something that you wouldn't normally wear. I rediscovered shorter skirts as my legs began to take shape. You might discover a feature that you've never noticed before and now's the time to play it up. Get in front of a three-way mirror and check out your changing/new body from every angle. Play dress up and try on colors, prints—move away from black and explore color. If you're currently wearing black, then at least throw splashes of color with it and add accessories that make you feel good inside. These small additions will definitely make all the difference in your outfit and mood.

19

Out with the Old

I had several clothes in my closet, some with tags still on them. I couldn't wait to get back in them or so I thought. Once I was able to wear these clothes, I noticed something had changed—me. I was no longer that person. As I lost the weight, I was doing some badly needed inner work. I was not only shedding weight, but I was also shedding old ideas and thoughts that no longer served who I was becoming. I made up my mind that I was no longer going to apologize for the light that came through me. Besides, on a lighter note, it was fun to shop again for new clothes. Although it might be more economical to hold on to those clothes, it won't do anything for you if you are not celebrating the new you with a new outfit. There might be a couple of key pieces that you'd like to hold on to, so pick and choose wisely what you want to keep and what you want to toss. The new you probably won't feel as comfortable hanging on to clothes that can no longer hold all that fabulousness anyway.

20

The Big Clean

Eating clean will save you a lot of grief while trying to lose weight. Clean eating basically means eating foods that are not processed or pre-packaged. This includes fresh fruits, vegetables, lean meats like fish and chicken. What it does not include: sugar, white bread and bad fats like hydrogenated and trans fat. Adopting this way of eating will do wonders for you and your physique. The weight loss program I followed did not allow much room for indulging in gravies and sauces that were usually ladened with fat. Most of the time I pretty much ate grilled chicken, fish and ground turkey alongside hefty portions of vegetables. I developed such an affinity for veggies that my mouth sometimes still waters when I'm in the produce section. I rarely order foods that look like they are swimming in sauce. This is where you can find a lot of your hidden calories. Keeping it simple while following a plan will help you reach your goals faster. Eating clean for the most part will help you maintain your weight loss goals. Save the sauces for special occasions after you lose weight and then use them sparingly. Be careful not to find a reason to make everyday a special occasion. Save those indulgences for birthdays, weddings, etc.

21

Send Them Packing

Don't allow your friends to make you stay in the past.
You are transforming on the outside, but you should
also be doing the inner work and transforming on the
inside. A former friend constantly reminded me of
things that I used to do. While her recollection made
me uncomfortable, I rarely said anything. This kind
of relationship went on for years until I finally took
a different approach and chose not to stand for it.
Ultimately, we had a disagreement about something
I did and in the process she started bringing up past
events to make her point. Rather than preserve this toxic
relationship, I chose to let it go. Listen, you are a divine
work in progress and you don't need anyone around you
to make you feel like a smash-up job. If you are going
to allow your friends to stick around, make sure they are
cheering you on your journey to your ever-evolving best
self and remember to return the favor. Isn't that what

Fit & Fab for Life

friends are for? If they are not treating you with kindness and respect, then send them packing and you keep on strutting as well. Don't let them weigh you down with old baggage you're releasing.

22

Can We Talk?

———◦◉◦———

Be open to talking about your struggles as well as your triumphs that you've experienced during your weight loss journey. People come up to me all the time and it's a blessing to share my story with the hope that it will help them on their journey. Winning this weight loss battle is somewhat of a struggle at times, but the rewards are well worth the sacrifice. We all have different ways of approaching this goal and talking about it helps us gather collective information that might be helpful in overcoming certain obstacles. I'm always inspired by others' continual journey to have the healthiest body possible as it motivates me, but more importantly it allows me to celebrate the success of others. I call them "weight loss rock stars." No two stories are alike and the fact remains that losing weight is tough and keeping it off is even harder. So, don't be afraid to open up and share as you will uncover new truths about yourself while helping someone else along the way.

23

It's a Family Affair

Can you hear Sly and the Family Stone singing in the background? This is what I thought about when I came up with this tip. But the truth is, we are all busy and chances are we have developed habits that are more or less reinforced through our families. Changing midstream sometimes rocks the boat and upsets the routine. As a result, you may be met with resistance from your spouse, your children or various other family members. Try to strike a balance between being firm and flexible. Modify recipes slightly and include your children in the process. Lovingly assure them that this is for the overall health of the family. Families can be one of the biggest saboteurs of your weight loss goals, but you have to be strategic in your approach with each individual. You have the final say on what goes in and out of your body. Sometimes you'll have to compromise and make a favorite family dish, but stick to your guns. Assure your spouse that they are not losing you, but instead gaining someone who is becoming more healthier so you can stay around a long time.

24

Cleaning Woman 101

Don't get me wrong, being a cleaning woman is a noble profession, but it's not one you should think about while at the gym. Whenever I go to the gym, I run into a lot of women who look like they are there to clean the gym. There are a few who even bring their own disinfectant to wipe off the equipment. Her look says, "let me get this done so I can go back to bed." Buying a couple of cute workout outfits will make you feel better about working out if you show up looking like you mean business. I'll admit I love workout clothes and even when I was heavier, I invested in a few pieces to make me feel good and look good in the process. You don't have to break the bank either. Stores like Target, T.J. Maxx have workout pieces that are inexpensive, but will help you look your best as you become your best. You can always give those pieces away. So leave the cleaning supplies at home and show up ready to work that body and look good doing it.

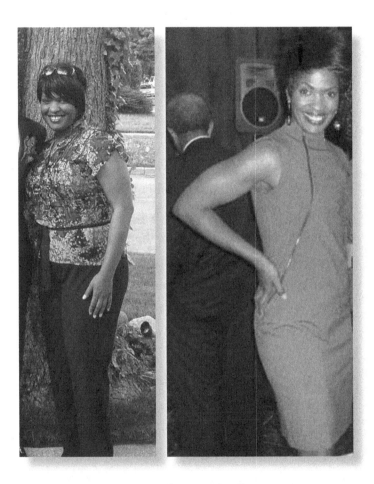

Me, Before and After

25

Test Drive a Trainer

———◦◉◦———

Everyone should have a trainer to learn how to properly use machines and do various exercises safely. It helps when you are first starting out so that you become less intimidated by the weight machines. If cost is an issue, work out an arrangement where you can split the cost with someone who is equally committed. Find a trainer who is willing to work with the arrangement and you are on your way. How long you use a trainer is entirely up to you. It's my job to look good on and off camera, so I retained a trainer long after I hit my weight loss goals. Sure I know how to use the machines and I could work out on my own, but keeping a trainer helps me stay accountable to someone, other than myself. So try out a couple of different trainers and find one who works for you because no one trainer fits all. It's a relationship and it should be a symbiotic one and not one where he or she feels sorry for you, but pushes you beyond where you think you are. Seeing my trainer on a regular basis kept the momentum going. Finding a trainer that will help you reach your goals is definitely worth the effort.

26

Play with Your Palate

———◈———

When you're changing your diet habits to lose weight, it is a perfect opportunity to try different foods. For example, I ate more fish and I experimented with various seasonings to add some pizzazz to everyday chicken dishes while losing weight. At one point, I thought I was going to burp feathers. Then I started eating more turkey burgers with grilled onions, and rainbow peppers to get my vegetable servings in. Try foods you wouldn't normally eat and break the monotony of chicken and fish. Playing with your palate gets your taste buds used to different foods. Try different condiments or add to light sauces to give them a different flavor. Eating doesn't have to be boring while you're losing weight. Instead of grilled chicken, try cubed chicken in a soup or topped over a baked potato with a ton of vegetables and creamy mushroom soup as a nice gravy. Cut up chicken and make a cherry almond chicken salad served with tiny wheat crackers or served on a wheat pita. If you're pressed for time, cook up some chicken breasts for the week. Buy a rotisserie chicken and make several meals for lunch and dinner. You can always add a dash of salt-free seasonings and throw some vegetables on the side.

27

Baby Your Body, Baby

What you put inside your body is important. Your body is your temple and it's the only one you have, so value it. Massages, salt scrubs, pedicures and manicures are numerous ways to appreciate your temple, head-to-toe. Taking time to love yourself enables you to become at peace with your flaws. I noticed the smaller I became, the more aware I became about various things I did not like about myself. It's not that I was down on myself, but I didn't like my narrow hips, but I loved my defined legs. So there was my tradeoff. Instead of focusing on this, I chose to focus on things that made me appreciate my efforts to become healthy. My strong shoulders and shapely biceps enabled me to not focus on the fact that I didn't have a six-pack that made you want to take a swig. Donna Karan said it best, "delete the negative, accentuate the positive." Sounds like

Francyne Walker

good advice to me and while you're at it, celebrate with a milk and honey scrub followed by a warm oil massage. You've worked hard and you've earned the right to generously pamper yourself.

28

Go Ahead and Have Fun!

Find extraordinary and ordinary ways to enjoy your life. Do karaoke, dance in the rain. There's a hilly area near my mom where every winter kids get their toboggans and slide down the hill. It doesn't matter how old you are, it just matters that you have fun. I've always wanted to go up in a hot air balloon, take up fencing, and learn capoiera. Sometimes it's the simple things that are so much fun like dancing with my niece. Going to the show with my son is one of the things I enjoy most. I also love having dinner with my family and allowing the love and laughter to flourish around the table. Did I mention I love to dance? Just do something that makes you laugh and makes you smile. It shouldn't necessarily revolve around food, but it's alright if it does sometimes. Just make sure it's a healthy meal that you and your family prepared. Preparing a new recipe with your girlfriends or significant other can be fun. Have a "fit and fab" party and invite a group of your friends over for a group training session with a hot trainer. Can you think of better motivation? Learning something different can be challenging and fun at the same time. When you're on your weight loss journey, you can fall into the trap of waiting until you've lost the weight to start having fun. Don't wait, have fun now by incorporating tiny moments of happy!

29

Keep the Blind Faith

There were days when I wasn't so crazy about working out, but I still kept my appointment with my trainer. I rarely cancelled because I was committed to my goals. Sometimes I would be so sore from the strenuous workouts and I would rub down with anything that would soothe the soreness. Despite the results coming slowly at first, I kept going to the gym. I huffed, puffed, lifted, grunted and even told my trainer a few times that I didn't like him. I was determined to keep working at it. Even after you reach your goals, you will have to continue working out. Sometimes we reach plateaus where it feels like the weight isn't coming off. Kick it up a notch; add another day of cardio, incorporate intervals or get some extra minutes on your favorite machine. Just don't give up, the weight will continue to fall off if you continue to work out and track your eating choices. Long after you've lost weight, you will have to continue working out even if you feel like it's not helping. Trust me, you don't want to see what happens when you give yourself a vacation too long to forget when you worked out last.

30

Do Some Inner Work

While I had lost the weight on the outside, I discovered there was some inner work that I needed to do. First, I had to silence my inner critic and be about the business of reaching my goals. This wasn't going to be an easy task, but it was important for me to acknowledge because I was an emotional eater. Knowing your triggers and deciphering them will help you respond differently. I know when I'm stressed, I reach for the cookies, cake and chips. Taking some "inner-ventory" and checking in with yourself is important. Journaling your thoughts, ideas and dreams is essential to getting what you want and eliminating what you don't want. This process takes courage and discipline, but the rewards of doing the inner work is worth it. Besides, it helps you get laser focus on what you need to do and be about the business of changing your situation. The added bonus of managing your emotions helps you manage your weight.

31

Reward Yourself Often

Celebrating your small victories along the way is highly recommended. It will help you reach the bigger goal. Say you have 30 pounds to lose. You would then break that up into smaller goals like one to two pounds a week. Do something for yourself that doesn't involve food as a reward. My girlfriend, Christie, used to do really cool stuff like skydiving or race car driving whenever she reached one of her weight loss goals. Ok, even if you're not that adventurous, do something special for yourself for every five pounds you lose. Your rewards should be something you're comfortable with. Maintaining your weight loss can be tough too, so reward yourself when you stay at your goal weight or when you exercise four to five times a week. Monthly or bi-weekly rewards will help you stay motivated and those tiny celebrations will give you a sense of accomplishment that you will want to experience over and over again.

32

Be Gentle and Loving

We all fall off the wagon sometimes on this weight loss journey. That's okay because LIFE happens. During my journey, I was sending my only son off to college and my mother was hospitalized for several months shortly after that. During that time, I stopped focusing on the kinds of foods I should have been eating. The great thing was I continued to work out on a regular basis despite ditching the diet plan I was following. This period lasted for about three months. Once everything quieted down, I resumed my program alongside working out. I didn't kick myself for the time I fell off the wagon. I have had my weight slide upward in the past and would sometimes feel really bad about it, but I realized this behavior was futile. We have to treat ourselves like our best friend and not always kick ourselves when we feel like we've done something wrong. I needed to remember how far I had come and celebrate that in the midst of my setback. I fell

Francyne Walker

off the wagon, but hey, at least I didn't break the wagon. But I moved on and went on to reach my goals. Stop crucifying yourself and congratulate yourself for making choices that bring about a healthier you! This is truly a journey, find what works for you and stick to it as much as possible.

33

Your Personal Best

———————◦❖◦———————

I can't tell you how many times I've heard people tell me not to lose too much weight. I went from a size 16 to a size 8, so the change was pretty drastic and it threw some people off. While some people didn't have a problem with the larger me, there were some people who thought I was getting too skinny. But that's just it, these people have nothing to do with my goals and why I choose to be a certain size. And trust me, whatever size you choose to be requires work to stay there for the most part. God bless those that don't have to work at losing weight or maintaining weight. Your personal best is personal and that's really all it is to it. You've worked hard and you're working hard to realize your weight loss goals. Don't let anyone deter you from that number. It's just a number that can be revised as you see fit. When I started at 215 pounds, 150 was the magic number, but it turned out that anything in the 155 to 160 pound range suited me just fine. I didn't panic because I didn't reach 150 as I realized my body just didn't feel right trying to slide closer to that number. I was happy with the way I felt and the way I looked. You are the only person who needs to be happy with your "personal best" goals.

34

Push Yourself Away

———⋄———

Staying at the table long after you've eaten is not a bad thing if you know how to stop going for seconds. Even while dining out, have them clear the table after you're done eating to avoid picking from your plate long after you're finished. If at all possible, split dessert or don't order anything at all. Learn to focus on something other than food like the conversation and spending time with a friend or loved one.

The holidays can be challenging, too, with all the buffet-style parties. Just determine how much you're going to eat and then get rid of the plate. Learn to eat until you're satisfied instead of being uncomfortably full. Moderation is key as it requires you to train yourself especially if you're used to eating double portions. Doing this will pay off big because you will begin to sense when to stop eating and not to overeat. Getting uncomfortably

Francyne Walker

full doesn't make the dining experience pleasant. Drink a lot of water before going out to dinner to alleviate getting too carried away at your meal. The full feeling will help you stop long before the "I need to unzip my pants" stage.

35

Make Play Dates

———◦◉◦———

Whether you're going out with your girlfriends or your special guy, you don't always have to go to dinner. Do stuff that's action-oriented and fun. Remember play dates were simply structured times to allow children to play together and give moms a chance to socialize. Structure dates where again, you take the focus off food. Sure, walking in the park might sound like a cheap date, but it will get you outside and moving. Doing active things engages you and gets the heart rate up. Activities like skating, Zumba and pole fitness classes are cool ways to bond with the girls or your boo. Just don't take him to the pole dancing classes! Think outside the box and have fun. Ballroom dancing and fencing classes are other novel ways to engage your body and mind while interacting with your friends. Incorporating new activities gives you a chance to try out new fitness activities. Why not hire a trainer to work out at home with you and several of your girlfriends? This is an inexpensive way to test drive a trainer and it beats the regular routine of going out to eat. Everyone can bring a healthy dish to share and it becomes one of the most healthiest play dates you can imagine. I always say camaraderie goes a long way whether you're losing weight or maintaining your weight.

36

Taking It to the Streets

Getting outside and taking in the fresh air does wonders to clear your mind. Provided your allergies don't start when you go outdoors, leaving the gym behind is a nice change of pace. A run along the river walk in Detroit or a fast-paced walk in Central Park, Belle Isle or any huge park can be just what the doctor ordered to get you out of the doldrums. Whether the sun is shining or the leaves are rustling in the wind, taking your workout outdoors will keep your fitness regimen interesting. Go with the flow of the season and take it to the streets or to the slopes. Find an outdoor activity that you love or would like to try and get moving. The activity can be as simple as walking or as elaborate as training outdoors for a marathon. Why not grab a bike and take it to the trails for a refreshing ride that will clear your mind and tone your thighs? Taking it to the streets will take your fitness to another level.

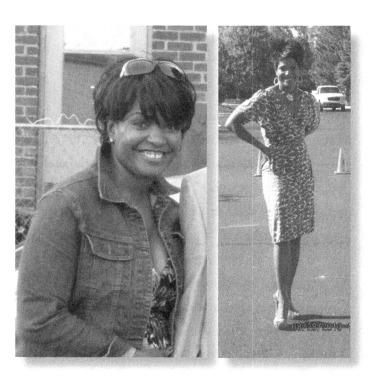

Me, Before and After

37

Choose Your Partner Wisely

Working out with someone is a great motivator, but you have to choose your partner wisely. You want to make sure you and your partner are committed to getting fit and staying fit for the long haul. It's helpful if you're both at similar fitness levels. This will eliminate feeling discouraged or acting as if you are in competition with one another. Sometimes it's alright to choose your spouse as your workout partner. You want to make sure you're working out as equals and that it doesn't turn into a personal trainer/client relationship. This should be an opportunity where both of you are encouraging each other. Make a pact with your workout partner to push each other when the other person feels like giving up. Integrity is the name of the game here. Pretend you're both running a marathon and you've promised each other that you won't let the other one give up until you both make it past the finish line. This is how it should

Francyne Walker

be when you decide to work out together. Don't let the other one quit. I've seen this kind or arrangement work out very well, but to thine ownself be true. If working out with someone else is not working out, then maybe your best workout partner is you.

38

The Sacred Place

I call the gym my sacred place. I know some might argue that the gym is a great place to meet the opposite sex, but if you find it hard to stay focused on your workout and a potential boo, at the same time, then eliminate the gym from that option. This is the place you come to work out and work it out. Don't ever sacrifice that to anyone. Of course, there are exceptions to every rule and if you have to meet that guy over on the weight machines, then always be in control so you never stop coming to the gym. At least work in a set and get your flirt on at the same time. This might seem extreme, but trust me you never want to get into a situation where you avoid going to the gym for stupid reasons and gain weight because of it. So make the gym your sacred place and make a commitment to yourself to work out and work it out there. Exercise is a great stress reliever so don't rob yourself of the one thing that can help you manage your stress. It's alright to be social, just don't let it get in the way of why you're there and what you're trying to accomplish. Keep it sacred and keep your focus. Even when guys step to you and try to talk to you while you're sweating and grunting on that elliptical trainer, be firm and polite. Don't get caught up working out with a guy either as this set-up can become inconsistent if feelings get involved. Hire a trainer who will not only keep you focused, but it will stave off unwanted interruptions during your precious workout time.

39

Now That's Stretching It

One should take a multi-pronged approach to fitness. In addition to cardiovascular strength and muscular strength, flexibility is important. Yoga, which incorporates slow and fluid moves of stretching and posing, not only improves your flexibility, but it clears your mind as well. There are so many forms of yoga and you should find one that suits you. Pilates is another great exercise that will improve your flexibility. These are floor mat exercises or reformers, where you perform the moves on machines. Warm-up stretches before engaging in any form of exercise are also helpful. This enables you to get your muscles warmed up so you're able to sustain moves. Don't disregard the importance of stretching. Hold your stretches instead of bouncing through them. Finishing up your workout with stretching while your muscles are still warm is good too.

40

Tweak if Necessary

Sometimes we begin a fitness regimen or nutritional program with the best intentions. You may start out with a commitment to walk for 30 minutes every day. With this routine, along with a sensible eating plan, it will help you lose your weight at a slow and healthy pace. However, our bodies become used to a routine pretty quickly. This may result in your weight loss efforts slowing down. The great news is that you can always tweak your routine as well as your diet to meet your goals. When my weight loss slowed down to a pound or two a week, I amped up my cardio routine by running three to four times a week. I averaged a weight loss of about three pounds a week once I did that. Writing down your food also helps you tweak your food intake by pinpointing foods that may be inhibiting your weight loss goals. Even after losing weight, you'll continue to tweak your workouts by adding new exercises and new recipes that will keep you motivated. Sometimes a little adjustment here or there is all you need to stay engaged while reaching your goals.

41

Become a Water Baby

Getting enough water will keep you from becoming dehydrated. A lot of people balk at the idea of drinking 64 ounces of water, but water fills you up and keeps you from overeating as it satiates hunger. If you find drinking water a challenge, then drink a glass in the morning. I take several supplements with water and then I follow with another glass of water. Carry a huge jug of water with you when you work out and be sure to finish it while you exercise. This is how I get the bulk of my water intake. A lot of times when I walk into the kitchen, I get a glass of water. Kick it up a notch, and drink alkaline water which can be purchased from any health food store. The health benefits are numerous. If you suffer from various diseases like diabetes or high blood pressure, be sure to check with your doctor before drinking alkaline water. Drinking water is the easiest step to take to having lifelong health. If the taste of water seems to make your taste buds go flat, then liven up your water with lemon, lime or orange slices. Throw in a few slices of cucumbers to give a refreshing new taste and get a vegetable serving in to boot.

42

Learn Something New

The great thing about fitness is that there are always new gadgets, new workout videos, and new exercises to try. I like learning new things. If you like working out in groups and you normally do Zumba, then take a boot camp class or a yoga class to give your fitness regimen variety. You will never know what you like and don't like until you try it. I loved the group camaraderie and the intensity of kickboxing classes. It allowed me to engage my mind and my body while Zumba enabled me to break a sweat and channel my inner sexy. Whatever your fancy, try it . . . and guess what? You don't have to stick with it forever. Just give yourself an allotted time to really give it a try. Courses are a good way to do this because it's built into your schedule like an appointment so you're even more likely to keep it. Check your local YWCA or community colleges and even your gym for some classes that will keep your fitness routine fun and challenging. Most of all, you will feel good on the inside for trying something new and mastering it. And the bonus? You'll look mahvelous on the outside dahling!

43

Pick Up Your Toys

———◆———

Remember the Thigh Master? Suzanne Somers made that one famous. How about the Ab Rocker? I like to call them "toys." Our mothers use to tell us to, "pick up your toys" now I'm telling you to pick up some toys. No, I don't mean Barbie dolls or Matchbox cars, I mean some fitness toys. If you walk around my place, I have a stability ball, resistance bands, hula hoop, and free weights. Even First Lady Michelle Obama hula-hoops which is actually kind of cool. These are occasional toys I use while I'm talking on the phone or watching television. Variety is the key in maintaining an active lifestyle hence maintaining your weight loss. These little fitness trinkets don't have to break the bank either. Go online to eBay because somebody is always looking to get rid of their stuff. Of course, it becomes your little treasure and you can incorporate these "toys" into your routine. My trainer would sometimes have me stand on a bosu ball for balance while lifting weights. The versatility of this little contraption was enormous. I could stand on the round side and then I would do push-ups on the flat side. Using some of these fitness gadgets are worth a try to help take your fitness level up a notch or add some variety.

44

Go Hard or Go Home

Everybody has an off day when they show up to the gym. Just don't make every day an off day. Long after I lost the weight, I retained a trainer to remain accountable and stay challenged. Some days I would show up and tell him that I just wasn't feeling it and he would invite me to go home. Of course, that was a challenge because I didn't quit that easily. Ironically, those workouts would be some of the best workouts leaving me refreshed and ready to conquer the world. I would feel my heart about to jump out of my chest at times during those sprints between sets, but it felt good to conquer my body and move past my comfort zone. If you don't know how to push yourself like that, then find someone who will make you "go hard" to help you stay in that zone. People used to wonder why I still had a trainer since I already knew what to do, but he kept me honest. He didn't listen to my whining or the grumblings under my breath and there were plenty times I did this. Sometimes all you have to do is just show up (well fed) and ready to work. Warm up for a longer period if you have to, but get in the game, go hard or go home. Fitness is work and it can also be fun. The rewards are so gratifying. Trust me!

45

Take Your Time

Every undertaking is a process and you shouldn't necessarily rush through it. If you're trying to lose weight for an event, be careful that you're not giving yourself an unrealistic time frame. Health and fitness is a life-long journey and while trying to fit into that dress and bikini by a certain date is great motivation, go beyond the event. Maybe you want to lose 30 pounds in a month, but I guarantee you if you make a life-long commitment with incremental goals along the way, you will lose 30 pounds in a realistic time frame. As I mentioned previously, I lost 60 pounds in approximately a year, including three months where I didn't follow my diet program. This was not my original goal, but I stuck with it because I was committed to the overall goal. Sometimes I find myself rushing through a set of a specific exercise and my trainer will remind me to slow down because working out is not a sprint, but a marathon. Set realistic goals, take your time getting there and "run" this marathon at your own pace, just look cute while you're doing it. Relish in your progress as you're making it.

46

Be Forever Grateful

You can't go wrong exercising an attitude of gratitude. No diet plan or workout plan can function without this necessary form of exercise. Having an attitude of gratitude is essential. Be grateful for who you are and where you are. It doesn't matter if you're a size 6 or a size 26, be grateful for your life and the ability to change your circumstances. I weighed 215 pounds at one point in my life, but I never lacked gratitude. I knew this was a temporary state for me and I was in control of my situation. Focusing on this fact made me grateful to be in a place to make a change. Your attitude determines your altitude—basically how high you want to go. If you count your blessings, they start to multiply right before your eyes. It won't take the weight off, but it will take the weight of the world off your shoulders temporarily. I was dealing with a sick parent while on my journey and it was stressful, but walking through that hospital I was always grateful. I didn't have to deal with the stress of a full-time job and the demands that a job would have placed on my time. Being grateful does wonders for your mind, body and soul.

47

Become a Spice Girl

·•⊛•·

A little bit of salt goes a long way, especially for those people who are salt-sensitive. I use very little salt and I can usually taste extreme amounts of salt in my food because I've trained my palate to eat alternate seasonings. I became a spice girl reaching for Mrs. Dash and a variety of other salt-free seasonings. Some foods are naturally higher in sodium so adding more salt sends you over your sodium intake. As an African American woman, I'm more diligent about my salt intake given the plethora of diseases I'm predisposed to such as diabetes, high blood pressure and hypertension. Alternate seasonings enable you to richly season your food without going overboard with the salt. Keep the shaker under control and use it sparingly. Now being a spice girl won't win you a Grammy or a spot on "Dancing with the Stars," but you'll score points in the healthy heart department keeping your sodium intake to a minimum. It's alright to use salt, but shake things up a bit and be aware of what your sodium intake should be and then act accordingly. Changing your salt intake will go a long way in guarding against diseases that are preventable.

48

Now, Don't Be Tripping

Traveling can test our best intentions to eat healthy. Processed foods, like salty nuts and sugary beverages on the plane, don't help. Hotels also pose their share of challenges, but you don't have to give into the temptation yet. If at all possible, pack your own fruits, unsalted nuts, and other healthy snacks to have on hand. Make your own trail mix and sprinkle it on some Greek yogurt for the trip. Having your own bag of healthy goodies will safeguard against the unhealthy temptations while "tripping." Just because you're on vacation abroad, doesn't mean your diet takes a vacation. Whether it's a business or pleasure trip, balance is certainly necessary and enjoying that exotic locale's indulgences should include healthy diet choices. Drinking plenty of bottled water is good and if you have to modify your exercise regimen, then do it. But don't do nothing. Even if it's 30 to 45 minutes on a treadmill or an elliptical trainer on a daily basis, make it count and do an interval set. This will get your metabolism buzzing during the set and long after you've finished. Walking through Tuscany is a great way to move your body while taking in the panoramic scenes. Jumping on a treadmill will help you wind down from a business meeting or a day full of convention programs. Keeping up with your fitness regimen will keep your indulgences in check.

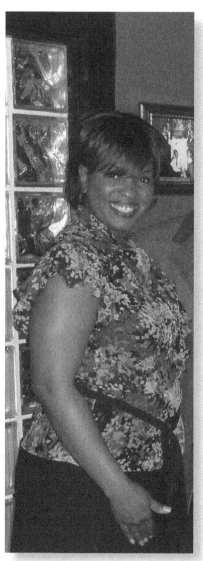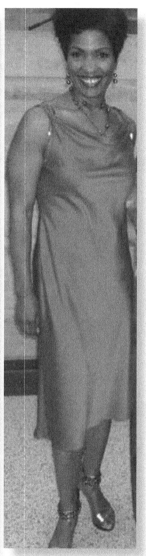

Me, Before and After

49

Celebrate Someone Else

———— ◦◉◦ ————

It's nothing more wonderful than celebrating someone who has reached their weight loss goals. Even while you're on your journey, congratulate and celebrate those who've gotten there before you. You have an idea what they've gone through and you can draw inspiration from them. Losing weight is not an easy task and maintaining weight loss is even more challenging. We're all in this together and collective encouragement goes a long way in keeping each other on point. Admiring someone who has already won the battle of the bulge is a great way to stay inspired. Adopt some of their habits that made them successful. You don't have to reinvent the wheel. You just have to get started and discover what works for you. A lot of weight loss programs have a built-in camaraderie and/or accountability system that ensures others are there to cheer you on in the small successes along your journey. Sometimes you'll come up against people who you cherish, like your friends and family, who comment that you're getting too skinny. Having others who support your success is essential to keep going on a sometimes long journey. So return the favor and celebrate someone else.

50

Above All Else, Value Yourself

I cannot emphasize it enough that this tip is the bedrock for all other tips to be fit and fabulous for life. While these other tips are certainly just as important above all else, love yourself. Exercising self-love puts you in the best shape of your life. Whenever I found myself in dead-end situations, whether it was a job, relationship, etc., it was my inner compass called "self-worth" that guided me out of those situations. I valued myself enough to want better and subsequently make the necessary changes to have what I wanted. That's the same thing with losing weight and even maintaining it. Whether you're a size six or a size 16, the value you place on yourself doesn't compare to all the weight you lose or gain. Honor your mind, body and soul. Surround yourself with people who do the same. Work to silence inner critics in your head (more importantly) and continue the work of becoming your best self. Recognize toxic situations and people so you can promptly remove yourself from these situations. Repeat after me: "This is me in all my splendor and it doesn't get any better than this." Say it and then say it again. Affirmations are invaluable to your well-being and are helpful in silencing your inner critics. Write them down, post them on your mirrors, post them on your ceiling and post them in your car. Create an affirmation tape that you play while you're sleeping. You are the most qualified architect when it comes to building and rebuilding you. Don't give that power to anyone else as no one can value you until you value yourself. Sure, we're cheering you on but you must become your own cheerleader when you're doing your best and even when you're feeling your worst. Create a "loved" life by simply loving yourself first, fully and deeply. Implement activities and ideas that you are passionate about. Value yourself enough to put those things first and then take care of everybody else. This is why I exercise in the morning as I developed that habit while my son was a baby. Working out in the morning enabled me to get it done and not have to worry about day-to-day interruptions that always inevitably cropped up. Whatever you choose to do, doesn't have to take away from you being a good parent, friend, spouse, etc. but carving out something for yourself will definitely make you a better person overall. And that's what being fit and fab for life is all about.

Acknowledgements

I am deeply grateful for the opportunity to inspire, uplift and show others how to get fit and be fabulous for life. This project could not have been possible if I had not had the courage to take this journey myself. I'm thankful for my family, my two sisters, Alison and Angela; my little fashionista niece Rayna; and my handsome and enormously talented son, Kevin. His ability to sit for hours and pour out his creative thoughts on paper inspired me to literally write "Fit and Fab for Life," on a yellow legal pad, while being stuck in an airport. I owe a special thanks to my son's father, Kevin Gilliam Sr. for his continual support and encouragement. Although my lovely mother will never get to read my first book, I trust she is guiding me from Heaven and I hope I make her proud. I am because she was. I'll love you forever Ma!

I'd like to also thank my friends who have cheered me along the way, especially Christie Taylor, Eve Walker and Cami Woods. The excellence of this project would not have been achieved without the help of another cheerleader friend, Skyla Thomas of Pleasant Words. Her proofreading and editing skills were invaluable. I am also grateful to the talented husband and wife team, Nate and Tameka Austin of NT Design Solutions. They took my crazy sketch for a book cover design and brought it to life. I have worked out with many great personal trainers over the years but I especially want to thank Glenn Lott for ignoring my whining and complaining to help me get in the best shape.

Additionally, I would like to acknowledge the most compassionate leaders you ever want to meet, my pastor, Dr. James L. Morman and his wife, Loretta Morman for always supporting me and allowing me to flow in my gifts for the past 8 years at Christian Tabernacle Church. Your prayers and covering have kept me during my best and worst times. I want to also thank all of my Facebook friends, Twitter and Instagram followers who inspire me to inspire them on a daily basis. I want to also thank each and every reader for embracing my words and applying them on a regularly basis to be fit and fab for life. Wherever we you are on your personal fitness journey, we are one and you are never alone. Thank you to Dr. Paula Thomas, who believed in me before I could finish the book, and bought the first copy of "Fit and Fab for Life."

A special thanks to all my writing instructors who helped me hone my gift over the years. I also want to acknowledge the inspiration of our First Lady of the United States, Michelle Obama, affectionately known as "FLOTUS." Thank you FLOTUS for providing a positive image in media for us to not just admire, but to look up to and be inspired to become our best selves. You are truly beautiful and you are "fit and fab for life" personified. I've got my sleeveless dress ready and I can't wait to meet you!

Lastly, I want to thank God for entrusting me with the gift to speak and write in a way that will move people to greatness. This has not always been an easy journey and I could not have done it without Him on my side. All things are possible and nothing is too hard for Him!

About the Author

Francyne Walker is a broadcast journalist, writer, motivational speaker, voiceover artist and an "accidental" actress. She is certified as a personal trainer through the International Sports Science Association. She has a B.A. in Journalism and an M.A. in Communications from Wayne State University. The self-proclaimed fashionista has one son in college and she currently lives the "fit and fab" life in Oakland County, Michigan.

Blog: For more information, read Francyne's blog, "Musings of a Slim Chick," on slimchick.wordpress.com.

Speaking for your business, church, organization: Francyne's presentations are funny, inspiring, motivational and filled with stories your audience won't soon forget. Read more about her keynotes and topics on the speaker page of the site. You can then book her directly or be referred to a speakers' bureau that represents her.

Website: To learn more about this author and when she'll be speaking in your area, please visit www.francynewalker.com.